KEGEL EXERCISE FOR FEMALE

ISAAC JONES

TABLE OF CONTENT

CHAPTER 1

INTRODUCTION

WHAT IS KEGEL

Before we go into the contest proper, firstly, you need to have an understanding on regarding the purpose of undergoing routine exercises and looking forward, on the efficiency on Kegel exercise.

Kindly note that Kegel is referred to as a standard of exercise that evolves the performance of a woman or female rather in strengthening the pelvic floor muscle, involving continual repetition of both sustained and swift contractions of the muscular system used especially to treat, eradicate, stop or end urinary self restrain or self control and improve one sexual functions.

CHAPTER 2

IMPORTANCE OF KEGEL EXERCISE IN THE BODY SYSTEM

There are a lot of factors to consider regarding the importance of kegel exercise in the body system, but we will go as far as explaining the most important aspects that will guide you to an effective wellness.

So many factors can weaken or hinder your pelvic floor muscle which include; undergoing surgical operation, childbirth, old age, excessive straining through constipation or uncontrollable coughing, and overweight etc.

There are further benefits of undergoing Kegel exercise which I will list below, it might sound awkward but it is necessary. They are;

If you are sneezing profusely, or coughing as the case may be, all you need do is take a few drops of urine and await the magic.

You will be so amazed at the impact it will do at that very instance.

Some women have asked severally if undergoing Kegel is cool to be done during pregnancy or after child birth, which is a YES.

Although, it is less helpful for women with urinary leakage when coughing, sneezing or either laughing, at such, you should avoid undergoing Kegel exercise if you discover you exhibit such ailment.

CHAPTER 3

HOW YOU SHOULD DO KEGEL EXERCISE

To undergo this practice is very easy as they are some basic factors you need to understand as you embark on the journey of strengthen your pelvic floor muscle;

To get started with:

Finding the right muscle: In order to discover your pelvic floor muscle, you need to take note of the following precaution, stop urination in midstream. When you've discovered this, you can undergo this practice in any position. But the best way or form I will suggest is undergoing such practice while lying down.

Rebrand your technique: To undergo this practice, try and imagine or picture yourself sitting firmly on a marble and tighten your pelvic muscles as though you are lifting the marble and stay focus. Do this for at a period of three seconds in an instant, then try relaxing at a countdown of three.

Keep up your focus: To desire excellent results, you need to focus on tightening just your pelvic floor muscles in your abdominal axis, buttocks, or thighs. Kindly keep away from holding your breath, instead to get the best result, breathe freely during this exercise.

Do a repeated action three times daily: It is at your best interest for you to attain the best result if you aim at repeating this actions at least three sets of ten to fifteen repeatedly a day.

More so, do not develop a habit of using this exercise to start and stop your urine stream. It is inappropriate for you to embark on this exercise while emptying your bladder could lead to an incomplete emptying of the bladder which can therefore increase the risk of urinary tracts infections in the body system.

CHAPTER 4

IT EFFICIENCY IN SEX AND PLEASURE

You will be amazed to know that this exercise can go a very long way in the aspect of your body system. If carried out effectively and consistently, it helps improve blood circulation in your vaginal and pelvic floor muscle, giving you an easier mode for you to reach your orgasm, increase in vaginal lubricant, relaxing your vaginal muscles. All this are what you will experience if only you carry out this exercise by following the methods I explained earlier.

CHAPTER 5

CAN KEGEL BE HARMFUL?

Several exercises are good for some other people but might not be good for some other people depending on their body structures. Going forward, kegel may be harmful to some people. Each pelvic floor exercises involving Kegel practice could help prevent or rather treat a complete host of pelvic floor disorders, from the urinary tract incontinence to prolapse. But it effectiveness and efficiency depends on your physical issues.

The issue might not be in the aspect of weakness but rather, over activity. According to research, it is true that pelvic floor dysfunction is often the result of muscle imbalance weakness or childbirth/injury, but not all the time. Pelvic floor dysfunction can also be regarded as very common in exercise instructors and elite athletes and most often not due to muscle weakness.

Most people that are experiencing such dysfunction mistakenly believe that the main cause of their problems is weakness, when the main cause of such dysfunction is majorly based on an overactive pelvic floor. It is such that an overactive pelvic floor can be turned on or contracted for too much time. If you are experiencing such, you should know that kegels exercise will likely worsen your symptoms or predispose you to develop symptoms if you are currently asymptomatic.

Kegel are extremely bad in this case and you should focus your attention on learning the teachings of a proper muscle control and muscle relaxation techniques using such exercise.

There are a lot of benefits from other treatments from the pelvic physiotherapist toolbox which include manual therapy in the form of an intense internal massage, as though as the teachings regarding pain, relaxation and activities to either avoid or modify.

CHAPTER 6

THINGS YOU SHOULD KNOW WHILE PERFORMING KEGEL

For a better performance and effective balance in undergoing this practice, it is best to know that when you are experiencing pains all over your abdomen or at your back after performing a kegel exercise, It is definitely a sign that you are not doing it correctly.

Always note that as you contract your pelvic muscles in your abdomen, buttocks, back and sides should remain loose.

More so, I will advice that you should not undergo kegel exercise excessively. If you overstress or work the muscle too hard, they will at a point become tired and unable to perform it necessary functions in the body system.

CHAPTER 7

DOES KEGEL INCREASE BLOOD FLOW?

You will be amazed at the length in which kegel exercise can do to your body if taken seriously. I know so many have been disturbed and wish to know if Kegel could increase blood flow, like is it possible. The answer is YES.

Kegel exercise as you may know is not just a regular exercise. This exercise could help you improve your erectile muscles and help you gain that control over urinary incontinence. This exercise does not only strengthen the erectile muscles but also increase blood flow in that area, in which an erection is depending on a constant flow of blood level strong enough to boost an erection and control enough to maintain it.

THE END